The Plant-Based Nutrition

*The Essential Guide to Plant-based
Nutrition with Tasty & Easy Recipes
for a Healthy Life and Losing
Weight Quickly*

Vegetarian Academy

The following Book is reproduced below with the goal of providing information that is as accurate and reliable as possible. Regardless, purchasing this Book can be seen as consent to the fact that both the publisher and the author of this book are in no way experts on the topics discussed within and that any recommendations or suggestions that are made herein are for entertainment purposes only. Professionals should be consulted as needed prior to undertaking any of the action endorsed herein.

This declaration is deemed fair and valid by both the American Bar Association and the Committee of Publishers Association and is legally binding throughout the United States.

Furthermore, the transmission, duplication, or reproduction of any of the following work including specific information will be considered an illegal act irrespective of if it is done electronically or in print. This extends to creating a secondary or tertiary copy of the work or a recorded copy and is only allowed with the express written consent from the Publisher. All additional right reserved.

The information in the following pages is broadly considered a truthful and accurate account of facts and as such, any inattention, use, or misuse of the information in question by the reader will render any resulting actions solely under their purview. There are no scenarios in which the publisher or the original author of this work can be in any fashion deemed liable for any hardship or damages that may befall them after undertaking information described herein.

Additionally, the information in the following pages is intended only for informational purposes and should thus be thought of as universal. As befitting its nature, it is presented without assurance regarding its prolonged validity or interim quality. Trademarks that are mentioned are done without written consent and can in no way be considered an endorsement from the trademark holder.

Tables of Contents

Why a Plant-Based Diet?

Why not? The health benefits associated with this diet make it one of the most highly recommended diet plans to follow.

The plant-based diet has very few restrictions, and it is not expensive to follow.

The meal plans are healthy, delicious, and good for your body.

The plant-based diet is high in fiber, water, and complex carbohydrates, which help the person to remain full for a longer period.

It is highly recommended for aged people, teenagers, nursing moms, and pregnant women.

A lot of research and evidence prove that it helps to lose weight effectively.

People who eat plant-based diets have low BMI, lower rates of heart disease, and lower cholesterol.

It is also effective in helping to prevent and manage diabetes.

Starting a Diet and Weight Loss

Starting a plant-based diet is easy: you do not need to eliminate huge food categories, and you do not need to subscribe to any expensive online plan. You need to follow these simple steps to get started with the diet plan:

Add more fruits and vegetables to your diet.

Start the day with a bowl of salad or soup.

Always cook a meal in oils that are plant-based like canola, olive oil, and peanut oil.

If you feel, need to munch on something, choose nuts and seeds for snacking.

For breakfast, choose tea and coffee that is unsweetened and without animal milk.

The meal should be comprised of those food items that are organic, whole, and full of vitamins, minerals, and protein.

You may add limited sweet treats. It's better to satisfy the sweet craving with fruit-based desserts and drinks.

It is highly recommended to only have 5-10% of the calories in your meal be from meat.

Try to include grain and legumes.

Choose your breakfast wisely by adding bread made with buckwheat, barley, or wheat.

"Go green" is the tagline for a vegan diet plan, and it is the best choice possible for healthy foods.

Advantages/benefits of Plant-Based Diet and Its Usefulness

- **Prevent hypertension**

The addition of healthy green vegetables, fruits, and healthy unprocessed food items contribute toward low blood pressure. When a person switches to a plant-based diet, it automatically reduces the blood pressure and increases the potassium. The potassium helps in lowering hypertension and anxiety. The nuts, legume, and grains provide vitamin b6 that helps to lower the blood pressure.

- **Effective weight loss**

Different research and study conduct that people following a plant-based diet tend to have a very low body mass index and have lower chances of getting obese. They also tend to have a very low rate of heart disease and diabetes. The plant-based diet plan is rich in fiber, protein, minerals, and calcium. All these nutrients make the body feel fuller for a longer period. It is one of the effective diets that treats obesity and reduces excess weight.

- **More energy and efficiency**

The food groups that are part of the plant-based diet are rich in good fats and nutrients that provide instant energy to the body and cutting down the meat; you can reap a lot of health benefits.

Lower the rate of cancer and cardiovascular diseases.

The good fat and omega 3 rich food help lower the fat. The whole foods plant-based diet improves the chances of avoiding cancer as we cut on red meat, smoking, and alcohol, and we all know all these items are a link to increased heart diseases.

Differences with Other Diets

- Vegetarian

A plant-based diet is totally different from a vegetarian diet. The main difference is that vegetarians eat some animal products such as honey and milk while a plant-based diet is exclusively made of plant products only.

- Vegan

There has often been some confusion as to whether the plant-based diet is just another word for veganism, or if they are a completely different concept with different rules, so let's go into that. There are many similarities between the two, but also some distinct differences. Are veganism and a plant-based diet the same thing? The short answer is no. The particular diet that is chosen and the label it is given depends on the individual, and the reason they have chosen to live this lifestyle. Many vegans choose to be so because they disagree with the slaughter and poor treatment of farm animals, and so they do not consume these foods. They also usually choose not to use leather or wear fur or any other animal products. Vegans do not eat any sort of meat, or product containing traces of meat. This includes any broths or ingredients such as gelatin. Vegans also do not eat any food products that contain ANY ingredient from an animal, including milk or honey. They do not eat any cheese, or yogurt, or margarine or butter, etc. Some slightly more hidden ingredients that contain animal products are whey and casein. These are all avoided. Vegans get most of their food from plant sources, but they are not strictly whole food plant based. They may not be as health conscious, and so many may choose to eat packaged and processed foods, yet stay away from those made of animals. This technically still falls within the parameter of their diet.

Plant-based folks eat a primarily plant derived diet- as close to nature as possible. But this does not mean that they are vegan, or even vegetarian. They may simply choose to eat mostly fruits, vegetables, nuts and legumes, etc. However, they may still choose to eat meat, and carefully choose meats that are antibiotics free, grass fed, and lived a free-range life. Many plant-based dieters believe that meat is still an integral part of a healthy diet, and so they just choose the best quality possible.

Whole food, plant-based diets usually take the qualities of both diets and even go a step further. Keeping foods whole refers to leaving them in their most natural state. So, vegetables and fruit are eaten as they are fresh, frozen or dried without preservatives or added flavor. Nuts are natural, without salt or sugar; grains are not refined or enriched or bleached. Most foods are prepared at home, or in a restaurant where the chefs share the same standards, as to not degrade any of the ingredients or take away any of their nutritional value. Many processed foods use what is known as plant fragments, rather than whole plants. They are reduced, or extracted or otherwise processed in some way.

Whatever the specifics of the diet someone chooses, if they tell you that they are vegan or plant based, you should assume that they do not consume any animal products at all, unless they mention it otherwise. This can help you to avoid accidentally serving them something that they will not be willing or able to eat. And feel free to ask someone about their diet, if you are curious. But make sure that they are willing to talk about it, and also that you listen with an open mind-not looking to judge or challenge their decision to adopt that particular diet.

- Pescatarian

The pescatarians adhere to a diet with seafood as the sole meat source. It is clearly different from a plant-based diet because it incorporates seafood and eggs dairy products, which are not part of the plant-based diet. Pescatarians cannot eat other meat apart from seafood.

- Flexitarian

A flexitarian usually eats a plant-based diet but occasionally adds meats to the diet. They are also known as semi-vegetarians.

- Fruitarian

This is a veganism subset and it mainly or fully consists of fruits, seeds and nuts. It does not include animal products. The difference with the plant-based diet is that fruitarianism only considers fruits and seeds while a plant-based diet considers other plants as food.

- Macrobiotic diet

This diet combines the concepts of principles of certain diets and spirituality of Buddhism to balance physical and spiritual wellness

The Plant-Based Food Group

Leaves

Leaf vegetables, or greens, are one of the most nutrient-dense foods you can eat. They contain plenty of vitamins (especially K, A, C, and folate) and minerals (like iron, magnesium, and potassium), as well as lots of chlorophyll, which is cleansing to the human system, particularly the liver. If you feel maxed out on salads, try adding some greens to a fruit smoothie or a soup. Puréed greens shrink quite a bit. The wide variety of leaves includes lettuce, kale, spinach, cabbage, Swiss chard, mizuna, arugula, bok choy, collard greens, mustard greens, dandelion greens, endive, escarole, watercress, sorrel, and tatsoi.

Roots

Root vegetables are generally made up of complex carbohydrates and starches. This is why they are usually cooked before being eaten, since cooking breaks down the starch molecules into easier-to-digest forms. However, carrots and radishes are commonly eaten raw in North America. The many root vegetables include carrot, beet, parsnip, rutabaga, turnip, sweet potato,

potato, celeriac, and radish. Many root vegetables, such as beets, radishes, and turnips, also have very tasty leaves.

Bulbs

This group includes onions, leeks, and garlic. Garlic's claim to fame is boosting cardiovascular health; it's been shown in many studies to reduce cholesterol, inhibit platelet aggregation (when platelets in the blood stick together, which is how clots form), and reduce blood pressure. Onions are also recommended for cardiovascular health, since they have sulfur compounds similar to the ones that make garlic so powerful.

Stems

Stem vegetables include asparagus, celery, and kohlrabi. They are all very nutritious green vegetables with very few calories. Kohlrabi is a relative of cabbage and broccoli, so it contains the powerful cancer-fighting and anti-inflammatory compounds of this family of vegetables.

Vines

Although some of these vegetables are botanically considered fruit, when it comes to nutrition and cooking, they are in the vegetable category. These vegetables have high water content and will shrink considerably when cooked. Because this category includes a variety of vegetables, they have very different nutritional profiles, but vine veggies are generally rich in carotenoids and vitamin C. Vine vegetables include zucchini, squash, eggplant, cucumber, peas, okra, tomato, and bell and hot peppers.

Flowers

Yes, flowers can also be vegetables! This group includes broccoli, cauliflower, and artichoke. Broccoli, as a dark green vegetable, is packed with nutrients and antioxidants. Although cauliflower has no color, it has similar nutrients and is just as good for you like broccoli.

Mushrooms

Mushrooms are not plants (they are fungi), but nutritionally they get lumped in with vegetables. The difference with mushrooms is that they eat organic matter and do not use photosynthesis like plants. Since they are a totally different organism than other vegetables, they have value in our diet by bringing in different nutrients, such as selenium and copper, as well as a powerful anti-inflammatory, cardioprotective, cancer-protective, and immune-supportive compounds. Mushrooms are high in minerals and protein per calorie and are also a good source of B vitamins.

Some of the mushrooms you might find in your local markets include chanterelle, shiitake, oyster, cremini, button, morel, and puffball. There are also many other types of edible mushrooms, including mushrooms used for their healing powers in Chinese medicine—some powerful enough to combat cancer.

Nuts and Seeds

1. Chia Seeds

   Chia seeds are amazing sources of vitamin C, protein, fiber, and calcium. They have to be soaked in liquid and allowed to expand. Once properly prepared, you can sprinkle them on top of almost anything!

2.Pumpkin Seeds

Pumpkin seeds work great for a tasty and easy snack and can also be added to salads, yogurt, and soups. They pack a lot of great nutrients like Vitamins C, E,

and K, omega-3 fatty acids, and iron in a small package.

3.Almonds

Commonly considered nuts, almonds are more accurately categorized as a fruit of the almond tree. They are wonderful sources of fiber, protein, magnesium, phosphorus, calcium, potassium, iron, and B vitamins. Like soybeans, they are often used in dairy substitutes and they have been shown to lower cholesterol, strengthen bones, and promote a healthy cardiovascular system. Plus, they are great for your skin and hair!

4.Flaxseeds

Flaxseeds are great additives to plant-based meals. They can be ground up and added to smoothies, oatmeal, cereal, or baked into muffins, bread, and cookies. They are high in protein, magnesium, zinc, and B vitamins. They also aid in digestion and help with weight loss by suppressing appetite.

5. Walnuts

These nuts are some of the best natural sources of omega-3 fatty acids. They also contain plenty of vitamin E, protein, calcium, zinc, and potassium. These, like many of the other nuts and seeds on this

list, can be enjoyed alone as a snack or added to other dishes.

6. Sesame Seeds

Sesame seeds are a great natural way to lower cholesterol and high blood pressure and can also help with afflictions like migraines, arthritis, and asthma. They are great in bread and crackers and can be used in stir-fry meals and salads.

7. Sunflower Seeds

These seeds are great for vitamin E and contain healthy fats, B vitamins, and iron. They can be eaten dry and are also used to make butter, a great alternative to dairy.

8. Cashews

Though cashews, like almonds, are not technically nuts and are rather the fruit of the cashew tree, they are most commonly treated as nuts. With their low sodium content and great flavor, they are a popular source of protein and vitamins.

9. Brazil Nuts

These delicious nuts from the Bertholletia excelsa tree mature inside a large coconut-like shell. They are wonderful for protein, fiber, iron, and many B-complex vitamins.

10. Pine Nuts

Pine nuts contain great antioxidants as well as lots of iron, magnesium, and potassium. They are low in calories and go wonderfully with many dishes. You can use them in baked foods or add them in sauces like an Italian pesto.

Legumes

1.Edamame

These cooked soybeans are not only delicious, but they also have an incredible amount of protein. In just one cup, a serving of edamame will give you 18 grams of protein. Look for the certified organic seal, though, because many soybeans in the United States are treated with pesticides or genetically modified. Edamame works great as a stand-alone snack or appetizer and can also be added into meals as a side or in a stir-fry.

2.Lentils

Easy to incorporate into almost any meal in a variety of forms, lentils provide an excellent source of low-calorie and high-fiber protein. They contain 9 grams of protein per half cup serving. They are also incredibly helpful in lowering cholesterol and promoting heart health. You can prepare them as a side dish, use them to make veggie burgers, substitute them for meat and make a delicious taco filling in a slow cooker or make a yummy dip with them.

3. Black Beans

Black beans are another vegetable like lentils that are wonderfully multi-use. They have great fiber, folate, potassium, and vitamin B6. They contain 7.6 grams of

protein in every serving and can be used to make anything from veggie burgers to vegan brownies. Imagine that!

4. Potatoes

Potatoes are a great, low-cost source of protein (4 grams per medium potato) and potassium. They're tasty and heart-healthy!

5. Spinach

One of the best green vegetables for protein (3 grams per serving), cooked spinach is an excellent addition to your plant-based diet.

6. Broccoli

When cooked, you get 2 grams per serving of this vegetable and also an excellent dose of fiber.

7.Brussels Sprouts

Another great green vegetable for protein, Brussels sprouts gives you 2 grams of protein per serving alongside a great deal of potassium and vitamin K. Be sure to get the fresh version, though, as they taste a whole lot better than the frozen kind!

8.Lima Beans

Containing 7.3 grams of protein per serving when cooked, lima beans make an amazing side dish or addition to a healthy salad. They also contain leucine, an amino acid that aids in muscle synthesis!

9.Peanuts and Peanut Butter

Widely recognized as a super food by meat-eaters and plant-based eaters alike, peanuts and peanut butter contain 7 grams of protein per serving and can be used in so many different ways. And who doesn't love a good childhood staple PB&J sandwich? Nearly all kinds of peanut butter are vegan, but keep a lookout for any that might contain honey if you are keeping strictly vegan and cutting out all animal products.

10.Chickpeas

Chickpeas are another versatile legume that can be prepared in a multitude of ways. Perhaps the most popular preparation is in the form of delicious hummus. With 6 grams of protein per serving, it'll be hard not to spread it on everything you eat!

Whole Grains

1.Quinoa

Quinoa certainly has made a splash onto the health food scene with countless people boasting about its beneficial qualities. Although it is actually a seed, we treat it mainly as a grain in the way in which it is prepared. This South American gem has an incredible amount of protein and omega-3 fatty acids and is an important staple of anyone looking to get more of these nutrients within a plant-based diet. It can be used in a multitude of dishes and is as versatile as it is healthy!

2.Wheat

A classic staple, whole wheat is incredibly beneficial to your health. Each serving of whole grain has about 2 to 3 grams of fiber, which is a great way to make sure your body is functioning healthily and properly. Be sure to steer clear of multi-grain, however, and go for the stuff marked 100% whole grain to make sure you are getting exactly what you need!

3. Oats

These whole grains are packed full of heart-healthy antioxidants. Oats are great and can be enjoyed as a fulfilling breakfast in the form of oatmeal and they can also be ground up and used as a healthier flour substitute when baking. Unsweetened oats are the best to buy and if you are craving a little something sugary, throw in a few berries or a dollop of honey if you wish.

4. Brown Rice

Brown rice is incredibly high in antioxidants and good vitamins. It is relative, white rice is far less beneficial as much of these healthy nutrients get destroyed during the process of milling. You can also opt for red and black rice or wild rice. The meal options for this healthy grain are limitless!

5.Rye

Rye is an amazing whole grain that contains four times the fiber of regular whole wheat and gives you almost 50% of day-to-day recommended iron intake. When shopping for rye, however, be sure to look for the whole rye marking as a lot of what is on the market is made with refined flour, thus cutting the benefits in half.

6.Barley

This whole grain is a miracle food for lowering high cholesterol. It can be quick-cooked like oats and serves as a delicious side dish. You can add whatever kind of toppings you desire to give it your own personal flair! Be sure again to seek out the whole-grain barley as other types may have the bran or germ removed.

7.Buckwheat

Buckwheat is a great gluten-free grain option for those with celiac disease or gluten intolerance. It's a great source of magnesium and manganese. Buckwheat is used to make delicious gluten free pancakes and easily becomes a morning staple!

8. Bulgur

This grain is a truly excellent source of iron and magnesium. It also contains a wonderful amount of protein and fiber with one cup containing about 75% of daily recommended fiber and 25% or daily recommended protein. It goes great in salads and soups and is easy to cook. Talk about amazing!

9. Couscous

This grain is another great source of fiber. A lot of the couscous you see in the store will be made from refined flour, though, so you must seek out the whole wheat kind so that you can get all the healthy, yummy benefits.

10. Corn

Whole corn is a fantastic source of phosphorus, magnesium, and B vitamins. It also promotes healthy digestion and contains heart-healthy antioxidants. It is important to seek out organic corn in order to bypass all of the genetically modified product that is out on the market.

Fruits

1.Avocado

Widely acknowledged as an incredibly beneficial and healthy super-fruit, avocados truly are miracle fruits. They are the best way possible to get the kind of substantial serving of healthy monounsaturated fatty acids that many people subscribing to a plant-based diet seek to supplement. They also contain about 20 different vitamins and minerals and are packed with important nutrients. On top of that, they taste amazing and go well with almost any dish, breakfast, lunch, or dinner!

2.Grapefruit

Grapefruits are packed full of Vitamin C, containing much more than oranges. Half a grapefruit provides you with almost 50% of your recommended daily vitamin C. It also gives you incredible levels of Vitamin A, fiber, and potassium. It can help with afflictions like arthritis and is a great remedy for oily skin.

3. Pineapple

This fruit can be prepared and enjoyed in a variety of ways making it not only a tasty and fun treat but also a great healthy choice! It is full of anti-inflammatory nutrients that can help reduce the risk of stroke or heart attack. Some studies show that it also increases fertility.

4. Blueberries

These little berries not only taste delicious and go with so many different dishes, but they are also full of vitamin C and healthful antioxidants. Studies also show that it promotes eye health and can slow macular degeneration, which causes older adults to go blind.

5. Pomegranate

Whether in juice form or seed, consuming pomegranate is a great way to get potassium. It has fantastic antioxidants (three times more than green tea or red wine) that work to promote cardiovascular and heart health as well as lower cholesterol levels

6. Apple

The old saying "an apple a day keeps the doctor away" is not just an old wife' tale! It is low-calorie and incredibly healthy. Apples contain antioxidants that protect brain cell health and are heart-healthy. They can also lower high cholesterol and aid in weight loss and healthy teeth.

7. Kiwi

This tart, delicious fruit is not only unique but also full of great vitamins like C and E. These are powerful antioxidants that some studies show help with eye health and can even lower the chances of cancer. They are low-calorie and very high in fiber. This makes them great for aiding in weight loss and they make a wonderful, quick, easy, and guilt-free snack.

8. Mango

Mangoes have excellent levels of the nutrient beta-carotene. The body converts this into Vitamin A which in turn strengthens bone health and the immune system. They also have a huge amount of Vitamin C-50% of the daily recommended value to be exact.

9. Lemons

Everyone knows that lemons and other citrus fruit are high in Vitamin C, however, they are also an excellent source of antioxidants, fiber, and folate. Lemons can help lower cholesterol, the risk of some kinds of cancer, and blood pressure. All at just 17 calories a serving!

10. Cranberries

Cranberries are another fruit that has more than one health benefit. They have great vitamin C and fiber levels and have more antioxidants than many other fruits and vegetables. At only 45 calories a serving, it is a great way to boost your immune system, keep your urinary tract healthy, and absorb other important nutrients like Vitamins E, K, and manganese.

Spices and Herbs

Spices and herbs are not only a way to add rich flavor to your dishes but they also have small amounts of important nutrients. A study of vegetarian males eating an Indian diet showed that they got between 3.9 and 7.9 percent of their essential amino acid requirements, along

with about 6 percent of calcium and 4 percent of iron, just from the seasonings in their food.

Many spices have protein, and although it doesn't amount to much in terms of grams, it provides a source of some of the amino acids that may be low in plant foods. Popular spices that will add a world of flavor to your food include cumin, coriander, cinnamon, paprika, and nutmeg.

Herbs like parsley, cilantro, mint, ginger, and basil pack loads of nutrients, and are most beneficial and flavorful when you eat them fresh. Parsley gives women 22 percent of their daily vitamin C recommendation, and men 27 percent, in just 4 tablespoons. All fresh herbs, like leafy greens, have a high antioxidant and chlorophyll content, providing energy and helping your body neutralize free radicals.

Nutrients in Plant-Based Diet

Carbohydrates

Some people worry about consuming too many carbohydrates by eating plant foods. Carbohydrates are your body's main source of energy and are completely healthy if you eat them in the form of whole foods (such as whole grains, vegetables, and fruit), since they contain lots of vitamins, minerals, antioxidants, water, and fiber. Fiber is also a carbohydrate, but its role is to facilitate digestion rather than give energy.

Whole grains and fruit have the highest levels of carbohydrates, with about 70 to 90 percent carbohydrate content. Eating a banana is an instant energy boost. The best food sources of fiber are psyllium or flaxseed and leafy green vegetables.

Protein

Protein can be found in all cells of the body. It helps to repair and build muscles, skin, bones, and the immune system. Protein is also needed to create hormones and enzymes, which are made up of amino acids. The body can make some of the amino acids but definitely not all of them. The ones the body can't make are called essential amino acids and must come from the foods you eat. Eating mostly plant-based foods can meet your body's daily protein needs.

Protein is an essential nutrient in the body. It not only helps in building and repairing muscles, but it also aids in maintaining our skin and bone health. The immune system also requires protein to function optimally in warding off diseases. So, if you are new to a vegan diet, you may have questions concerning your protein sources. Of course, this is attributed to the myth that plant-based diets don't provide the body with sufficient nutrients.

However, several plant foods will provide you with the protein you need in your diet. Some of these foods include beans, soy products, seeds, nuts, peas, vegetables, and whole grains. When looking for proteins in vegetables, your shopping cart should be filled with veggies like broccoli, yellow sweet corn, potatoes, lentils, green peas, Brussels sprouts, broccoli rabe, avocado, and cauliflower.

Evidently, you can see that you have plenty of options to choose from when in search of protein in your diet. Now, let's do some math to determine the amount of protein you might need in your diet. According to the Dietary

Reference Intakes, the amount of protein you should consume daily is equivalent to 0.8 grams per kilogram of your body weight, or 0.36 grams per pound. Say you weigh 80 kilograms. You should multiply this by 0.8 grams to determine the protein quantity you require daily. In this case, the quantity of protein will be 64 grams.

The various foods mentioned above offer varying amounts of protein. This implies that combining several veggies together will provide you with what you need. A one cup serving of lentils, for instance, will provide you with 18 grams of protein. A cup of green peas, on the other hand, will only provide you with 8.5 grams of protein. Judging from the numbers, all you need is a mix of different plant foods to meet your daily protein intake.

Fats

Your body needs enough dietary fat to function, maintain metabolism, and absorb and utilize minerals and certain vitamins. People with cold hands and feet, amenorrhea (missed menstrual periods), or dry skin, hair, or throat may need more fats in their diet, and particularly saturated fats like coconut oil. To be clear, eating healthy fat in reasonable amounts doesn't make you fat.

Oils are 100 percent fat and aren't something you necessarily need to eat, but they are great for carrying rich flavor and mouthfeel in a dish, particularly when you're transitioning to a healthier diet. If you use oils, it's best to keep them minimal and use unrefined oils like olive, coconut, sesame, and avocado. (Refined oils include canola, soy, sunflower, and corn oil.) You can easily sauté vegetables for two people with just a teaspoon of oil.

That doesn't mean you should never eat oils, though, and some people can actually benefit from concentrated fats. For example, flax oil or concentrated DHA might be necessary for someone with issues digesting and utilizing omega-3 fatty acids.

Omega-3 fatty acids are also essential nutrients, meaning that the body cannot produce them. There are three forms of omega-3 fatty acids:

Docosahexaenoic acid (DHA)

Alpha-linolenic acid (ALA)

Eicosapentaenoic acid (EPA)

Individuals who eat fish usually obtain DHA and EPA. ALA, on the other hand, is obtained from plant foods. The good news is that the body can convert ALA obtained from plants into DHA and EPA. However, the process is not as efficient. Consequently, you could supplement your diet with hemp seed oil, flaxseed oil, or chia seeds to aid in optimizing the conversion process.

Other recommended foods to ingest include algal oil, walnuts, perilla oil, and Brussels sprouts.

The information detailed in this section should help you realize that important nutrients that are often assumed to be present only in animal products can also be obtained from plant foods. Therefore, knowing and understanding the nutrients you are getting from your plant foods is important; it confirms that you are getting all the vital nutrients your body requires for optimal functioning.

Vitamin C

Vitamin C will be an easier nutrient to obtain since most fruits and vegetables can provide the body with this vital nutrient. This vitamin helps in strengthening the body's immune system. As a result, vitamin C is often perceived as a remedy for the common cold. Recommended vegan foods to add to your diet here include broccoli, pineapple, Brussels.

Recipes

Fruity Granola

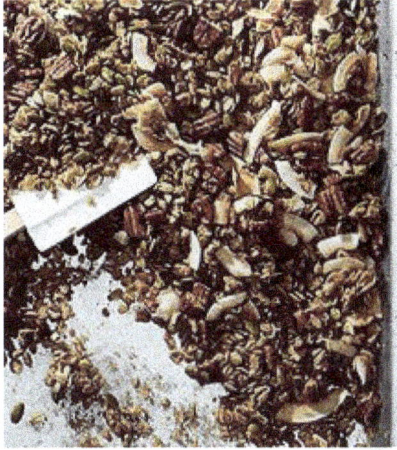

Preparation Time: 15 Minutes

Cooking Time: 45 Minutes

Servings: 5

Ingredients

- 2 cups rolled oats
- ¾ cup whole-wheat flour
- 1 tablespoon ground cinnamon
- 1 teaspoon ground ginger (optional)
- ½ cup sunflower seeds, or walnuts, chopped

- ½ cup almonds, chopped
- ½ cup pumpkin seeds
- ½ cup unsweetened shredded coconut
- 1¼ cups pure fruit juice (cranberry, apple, or something similar)
- ½ cup raisins, or dried cranberries
- ½ cup goji berries (optional)

Directions

1. Preheat the oven to 350°F.
2. Mix together the oats, flour, cinnamon, ginger, sunflower seeds, almonds, pumpkin seeds, and coconut in a large bowl.
3. Sprinkle the juice over the mixture, and stir until it's just moistened. You might need a bit more or a bit less liquid, depending on how much your oats and flour absorb.
4. Spread the granola on a large baking sheet (the more spread out it is the better), and put it in the oven. After about 15 minutes, use a spatula to turn the granola so that the middle gets dried out. Let the granola bake until it's as crunchy as you want it, about 30 minutes more.

5. Take the granola out of the oven and stir in the raisins and goji berries (if using). Store leftovers in an airtight container for up to 2 weeks.

6. Serve with non-dairy milk and fresh fruit, use as a topper for morning porridge or a smoothie bowl to add a bit of crunch, or make a granola parfait by layering with non-dairy yogurt or puréed banana.

Per Serving (½ cup)
Calories: 398; Protein: 11g; Total fat: 25g; Carbohydrates: 39g; Fiber: 8g

Pumpkin Steel-Cut Oats

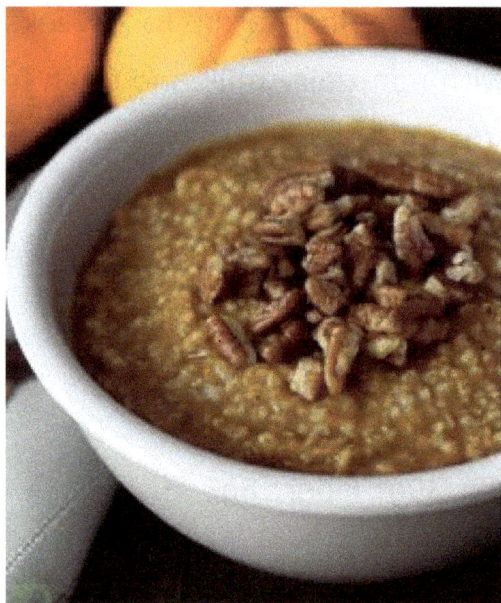

Preparation Time: 2 Minutes

Cooking Time: 35 Minutes

Servings: 4

Ingredients

3 cups water

- 1 cup steel-cut oats
- ½ cup canned pumpkin purée
- ¼ cup pumpkin seeds (pepitas)
- 2 tablespoons maple syrup
- Pinch salt

Directions

1. In a large saucepan, bring the water to a boil.
2. Add the oats, stir, and reduce the heat to low. Simmer until the oats are soft, 20 to 30 minutes, continuing to stir occasionally.
3. Stir in the pumpkin purée and continue cooking on low for 3 to 5 minutes longer. Stir in the pumpkin seeds and maple syrup, and season with the salt.

4. Divide the oatmeal into 4 single-serving containers. Let cool before sealing the lids.
5. Place the airtight containers in the refrigerator for 5 days or freeze for up to 3 months. To thaw, refrigerate overnight. Reheat in the microwave for 2½ minutes or in a skillet over medium-high heat for 6 to 8 minutes.

Nutrition: Calories:121; Protein: 4g; Total fat: 5g; Carbohydrates: 17g; Fiber: 2g

Granola

PREPARATION TIME: 5 MINUTES

Cooking Time: 15 MINUTES

Servings: about 8 cups

Ingredients

- 51/2 cups old-fashioned oats
- 11/2 cups slivered almonds
- 1/2 cup shelled sunflower seeds
- 1 cup golden raisins
- 1 cup shredded unsweetened coconut
- 1 cup pure maple syrup
- 1/2 teaspoon ground cinnamon
- 1/4 teaspoon ground allspice
- Pinch salt

Directions

1. Preheat the oven to 325°F. Spread the oats, almonds, and sunflower seeds in a 9 x 13-inch baking pan and place in the oven for 10 minutes.
2. Remove from the oven and reduce the temperature to 300°F. Add the raisins, coconut,

maple syrup, cinnamon, allspice, and salt and stir to combine.

3. Return the pan to the oven and bake for 15 minutes, or until the mixture is crisp and dry. Be careful not to burn.

4. Remove from oven and let cool completely, 30 minutes. Transfer to an airtight container and store in the refrigerator where it will keep for several weeks.

Chocolate Quinoa Breakfast Bowl

Preparation Time: 5 Minutes

Cooking Time: 30 Minutes

Servings: 2

Ingredients

- 1 cup quinoa
- 1 teaspoon ground cinnamon
- 1 cup non-dairy milk
- 1 cup water
- 1 large banana
- 2 to 3 tablespoons unsweetened cocoa powder, or carob
- 1 to 2 tablespoons almond butter, or other nut or seed butter
- 1 tablespoon ground flaxseed, or chia or hemp seeds
- 2 tablespoons walnuts
- ¼ cup raspberries

Directions

1. Put the quinoa, cinnamon, milk, and water in a medium pot. Bring to a boil over high heat, then turn down low and simmer, covered, for 25 to 30 minutes.

2. While the quinoa is simmering, purée or mash the banana in a medium bowl and stir in the cocoa powder, almond butter, and flaxseed.

3. To serve, spoon 1 cup cooked quinoa into a bowl, top with half the pudding and half the walnuts and raspberries.

4.

Nutrition: Calories: 392; Protein: 12g; Total fat: 19g; Saturated fat: 1g; Carbohydrates: 49g; Fiber: 10g

Savory Oatmeal Porridge

Preparation Time: 2 Minutes

Cooking Time: 25 Minutes

Servings: 4

Ingredients

- 2½ cups vegetable broth
- 2½ cups unsweetened almond milk or other plant-based milk
- ½ cup steel-cut oats
- 1 tablespoon farro
- ½ cup slivered almonds
- ¼ cup nutritional yeast
- 2 cups old-fashioned rolled oats
- ½ teaspoon salt (optional)
-

Directions

1. In a large saucepan or pot, bring the broth and almond milk to a boil. Add the oats, farro, almond slivers, and nutritional yeast. Cook over medium-high heat for 20 minutes, stirring occasionally.
2. Add the rolled oats and cook for another 5 minutes, until creamy. Stir in the salt (if using).

3. Divide into 4 single-serving containers.

4. Let cool before sealing the lids. Place the airtight containers in the refrigerator for 5 days or freeze for up to 3 months. To thaw, refrigerate overnight. Reheat in the microwave for 2½ minutes or in a skillet over medium-high heat for 6 to 8 minutes.

Nutrition: Calories: 208; Protein: 14g; Total fat: 8g; Saturated fat: 1g; Carbohydrates: 22g; Fiber: 7g

Muesli and Berries Bowl

Preparation Time: 10 Minutes

Cooking Time: 0 Minutes

Servings: 5

Ingredients

FOR THE MUESLI

- 1 cup rolled oats
- 1 cup spelt flakes, or quinoa flakes, or more rolled oats
- 2 cups puffed cereal
- ¼ cup sunflower seeds
- ¼ cup almonds
- ¼ cup raisins
- ¼ cup dried cranberries
- ¼ cup chopped dried figs
- ¼ cup unsweetened shredded coconut
- ¼ cup non-dairy chocolate chips
- 1 to 3 teaspoons ground cinnamon

FOR THE BOWL

- ½ cup non-dairy milk, or unsweetened applesauce
- ¾ cup muesli
- ½ cup berries

Directions

Put the muesli ingredients in a container or bag and shake.

Combine the muesli and bowl ingredients in a bowl or to-go container.

Substitutions: Try chopped Brazil nuts, peanuts, dried cranberries, dried blueberries, dried mango, or whatever inspires you. Ginger and cardamom are interesting flavors if you want to branch out on spices.

Nutrition: Calories: 441; Protein: 10g; Total fat: 20g; Carbohydrates: 63g; Fiber: 13g

Breakfast Casserole

Preparation Time: 15 Minutes

Cooking Time: 0 Minutes

Servings: 6 Servings

Ingredients

- 1 cup quick-cooking grits
- 1/2 cup shredded vegan Cheddar cheese
- 2 tablespoons vegan margarine
- 1 cup cooked and chopped tempeh bacon or vegan sausage
- 1 cup fresh or frozen corn kernels

Directions

1. Preheat the oven to 375°F. Lightly oil a 9 x 13-inch baking pan and set aside.
2. In a large saucepan, combine the soy milk and broth and bring to a boil over high heat. Add salt to taste (depending on the saltiness of your broth) and stir in the grits. Reduce the heat to low and cook, stirring occasionally, until the grits are

thickened but not stiff. Turn off the heat and stir in the cheese, margarine, tempeh bacon, and corn.

3. Scrape the mixture into the prepared baking pan. Spread evenly, smooth the top, and bake until slightly puffed and golden brown, about 45 minutes. Serve immediately.

Cinnamon And Spice Overnight Oats

PREPARATION TIME: 10 MINUTES • OVERNIGHT TO SOAK

Servings: 5

Ingredients

- 2½ cups old-fashioned rolled oats
- 5 tablespoons pumpkin seeds (pepitas)
- 5 tablespoons chopped pecans
- 5 cups unsweetened plant-based milk
- 2½ teaspoons maple syrup or agave syrup
- ½ to 1 teaspoon salt
- ½ to 1 teaspoon ground cinnamon
- ½ to 1 teaspoon ground ginger
- Fresh fruit (optional)
-

Directions

Line up 5 wide-mouth pint jars. In each jar, combine ½ cup of oats, 1 tablespoon of pumpkin seeds, 1 tablespoon of pecans, 1 cup of plant-based milk, ½ teaspoon of maple syrup, 1 pinch of salt, 1 pinch of cinnamon, and 1 pinch of ginger.

Stir the ingredients in each jar. Close the jars tightly with lids. To serve, top with fresh fruit (if using). Place the airtight jars in the refrigerator at least overnight before eating and for up to 5 days.

Nutrition: Calories:177; Protein: 6g; Total fat: 9g; Carbohydrates: 19g; Fiber: 4g

Baked Banana French Toast with Raspberry Syrup

Preparation Time: 10 Minutes

Cooking Time: 30 Minutes

Servings: 8 Slices

Ingredients

FOR THE FRENCH TOAST

1 banana

1 cup coconut milk

1 teaspoon pure vanilla extract

¼ teaspoon ground nutmeg

½ teaspoon ground cinnamon

1½ teaspoons arrowroot powder

Pinch sea salt

8 slices whole-grain bread

FOR THE RASPBERRY SYRUP

1 cup fresh or frozen raspberries, or other berries

2 tablespoons water, or pure fruit juice

1 to 2 tablespoons maple syrup, or coconut sugar (optional)

Directions

1. Preheat the oven to 350°F.

2. In a shallow bowl, purée or mash the banana well. Mix in the coconut milk, vanilla, nutmeg, cinnamon, arrowroot, and salt.

3. Dip the slices of bread in the banana mixture, and then lay them out in a 13-by-9-inch baking dish. They should cover the bottom of the dish and can overlap a bit but shouldn't be stacked on top of each other. Pour any leftover banana mixture over the bread, and put the dish in the oven.

4. Bake about 30 minutes, or until the tops are lightly browned.

5. Serve topped with raspberry syrup.

6. To Make the Raspberry Syrup

7. Heat the raspberries in a small pot with the water and the maple syrup (if using) on medium heat.

8. Leave to simmer, stirring occasionally and breaking up the berries, for 15 to 20 minutes, until the liquid has reduced.

9. Leftover raspberry syrup makes a great topping for simple oatmeal as a quick and delicious breakfast, or as a drizzle on top of whole-grain toast smeared with natural peanut butter.

Nutrition: Calories: 166; Protein: 5g; Total fat: 7g; Saturated fat: 1g; Carbohydrates: 23g;

Great Green Smoothie

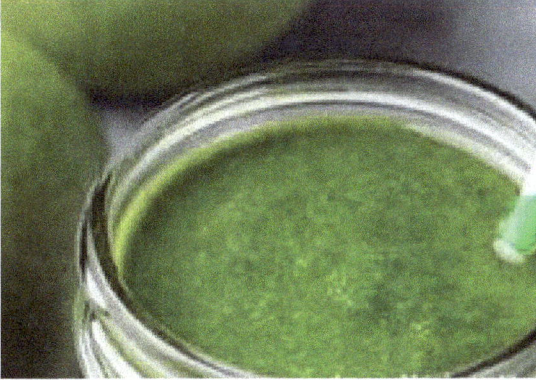

Preparation Time: 5 Minutes

Cooking Time: 0 Minutes

Servings: 4

Ingredients

- 4 bananas, peeled
- 4 cups hulled strawberries
- 4 cups spinach
- 4 cups plant-based milk
-

Directions

1. Open 4 quart-size, freezer-safe bags. In each, layer in the following order: 1 banana (halved or

sliced), 1 cup of strawberries, and 1 cup of spinach. Seal and place in the freezer.

2. To serve, take a frozen bag of Great Green Smoothie ingredients and transfer to a blender. Add 1 cup of plant-based milk, and blend until smooth. Place freezer bags in the freezer for up to 2 months.

Nutrition: Calories: 173; Protein: 4g; Total fat: 2g; Carbohydrates: 40g; Fiber: 7g

Summer Harvest Pizza

Preparation Time: 20 minutes

Cooking Time: 15 minutes

Servings: 2

Ingredients:

- 1 Lavash flatbread, whole grain
- 4 Tbsp Feta spread, store-bought
- ½ cup cheddar cheese, shredded
- ½ cup corn kernels, cooked
- ½ cup beans, cooked
- ½ cup fire-roasted red peppers, chopped
-

Directions:

1. Preheat oven to 350ºF.
2. Cut Lavash into two halves. Bake crusts on a pan in the oven for 5 minutes.
3. Spread feta spread on both crusts. Top with remaining ingredients.
4. Bake for another 10 minutes.

Nutrition:

Calories 230

Carbohydrates 23 g

Fats 15 g

Protein 11 g

Whole Wheat Pizza with Summer Produce

Preparation Time: 15 minutes

Cooking Time: 15 minutes

Servings: 2

Ingredients:

- 1 pound whole wheat pizza dough
- 4 ounces goat cheese
- 2/3 cup blueberries
- 2 ears corn, husked
- 2 yellow squash, sliced
- 2 Tbsp olive oil

Directions:

1. Preheat the oven to 450°F.
2. Roll the dough out to make a pizza crust.
3. Crumble the cheese on the crust. Spread remaining ingredients, then drizzle with olive oil.
4. Bake for about 15 minutes. Serve.

Nutrition:

Calories 470

Carbohydrates 66 g

Fats 18 g

Protein 17 g

Spicy Chickpeas

Preparation Time: 15 minutes

Cooking Time: 20 minutes

Servings: 8

Ingredients:

- 1 Tbsp extra-virgin olive oil
- 1 yellow onion, diced
- 1 tsp curry
- ¼ tsp allspice
- 1 can diced tomatoes
- 2 cans chickpeas, rinsed, drained
- Salt, cayenne pepper, to taste

Directions:

1. Simmer onions in 1 Tbsp oil for 4 minutes.
2. Add allspice and pepper, cook for 2 minutes.
3. Stir in tomatoes, and cook for another 2 minutes.
4. Add chickpeas, and simmer for 10 minutes.
5. Season with salt, and serve.

Nutrition:

Calories 146

Carbohydrates 25 g

Fats 3 g

Protein 5 g

Farro with Pistachios & Herbs

Preparation Time: 20 minutes

Cooking Time: 45 minutes

Servings: 10

Ingredients:

- 2 cups farro
- 4 cups water
- 1 tsp kosher salt, divided
- 2½ Tbsp extra-virgin olive oil
- 1 onion, chopped
- 2 cloves garlic, minced
- ½ tsp ground pepper, divided
- ½ cup parsley, chopped
- 4 oz salted shelled pistachios, toasted, chopped

Directions:

1. Combine farro, water, and ¾ tsp salt, simmer for 40 minutes.
2. Cook onion and garlic in 2 Tbsp oil for 5 minutes.
3. Combine ½ tsp oil, ¼ tsp pepper, parsley, pistachios, and toss well.
4. Combine all. Season with salt and pepper.

Nutrition:

Calories 220

Carbohydrates 30 g

Fats 9 g

Protein 8 g

Millet and Teff with Squash & Onions

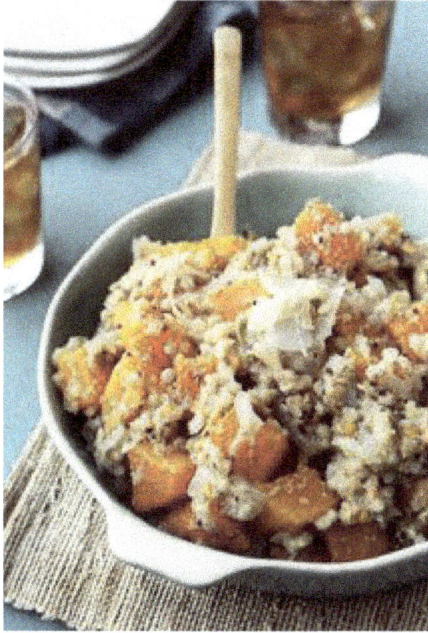

Preparation Time: 10 minutes

Cooking Time: 20 minutes

Servings: 6

Ingredients:

- 1 cup millet
- ½ cup teff grain
- 4½ cups of water
- 1 onion, sliced
- 1 butternut squash, chopped
- Sea salt, to taste

Directions:

1. Rinse millet, and put in a large pot.

2. Add remaining ingredients. Mix well.

3. Simmer 20 minutes until all the water is absorbed.

4. Serve hot.

Nutrition:

Calories 200

Carbohydrates 40 g

Fats 2 g

Protein 6 g

Brown Rice Tabbouleh

Preparation Time: 20 minutes

Cooking Time: 0 minutes

Servings: 6

Ingredients:

- 3 cups brown rice, cooked
- ¾ cup cucumber, chopped
- ¾ cup tomato, chopped
- ¼ cup mint leaves, chopped
- ¼ cup green onions, sliced
- ¼ cup olive oil
- ¼ cup lemon juice
- Salt, pepper, to taste

Directions:

1. Combine all ingredients in a large bowl.
2. Toss well and chill for 20 min.

Nutrition:

Calories 201

Carbohydrates 25 g

Fats 10 g

Protein 3 g

Healthy Hoppin' John

Preparation Time: 15 minutes

Cooking Time: 1 hour

Servings: 4

Ingredients:

- 1 Tbsp extra-virgin olive oil
- 1 onion, diced
- 2 garlic cloves, minced
- 1 cup of dried black-eyed peas
- 1 cup brown rice, uncooked
- 4 cups water
- Salt, pepper, to taste

Directions:

1. Cook the onions and garlic in oil for 3 minutes.
2. Combine the peas, salt, brown rice, and 4 cups of water and bring to a boil.
3. Add pepper. Simmer for 45 minutes.
4. Serve hot.

Nutrition:

Calories 248

Carbohydrates 47 g

Fats 5 g

Protein 6 g

Beans & Greens Bowl

Preparation Time: 2 minutes

Cooking Time: 2 minutes

Servings: 1

Ingredients:

- 1½ cups curly kale, washed, chopped
- ½ cup black beans, cooked
- ½ avocado
- 2 Tbsp feta cheese, crumbled
-

Directions:

1. Mix the kale and black beans in a microwavable bowl and heat for about 1 ½ minute.
2. Add the avocado and stir well. Top with feta.

Nutrition:

Calories 340

Carbohydrates 32 g

Fats 19 g

Protein 13 g

Black Beans & Brown Rice

Preparation Time: 2 minutes

Cooking Time: 45 minutes

Servings: 4

Ingredients:

- 4 cups water
- 2 cups brown rice, uncooked
- 1 can no-salt black beans
- 3 cloves garlic, minced

Directions:

1. Bring the water and rice to boil, simmer for 40 minutes.
2. In a pan, cook the black beans with their liquid and the garlic for 5 minutes.
3. Toss the rice and beans together, and serve.

Nutrition:

Calories 220

Carbohydrates 45 g

Fats 1.5 g

Protein 7 g

Yucatan Bean & Pumpkin Seed Appetizer

Preparation Time: 10 minutes

Cooking Time: 3 minutes

Servings: 8

Ingredients:

- ¼ cup pumpkin seeds
- 1 can white beans
- 1 tomato, chopped
- 1/3 cup onion, chopped
- 1/3 cup cilantro, chopped
- 4 Tbsp lime juice
- Salt, pepper, to taste

Directions:

1. Toast the pumpkin seeds for 3 minutes to lightly brown. Let cool, and then chop in a food processor.
2. Mix in the remaining ingredients. Season with salt and pepper, and serve.

Nutrition:

Calories 12 g

Fats 2 g

Carbohydrates 12 g

Protein 5 g

Butter Bean Hummus

Preparation Time: 5 minutes

Cooking Time: 0 minutes

Servings: 4

Ingredients:

- 1 can butter beans, drained, rinsed
- 2 garlic cloves, minced
- ½ lemon, juiced
- 1 Tbsp olive oil
- 4 sprigs of parsley, minced
- Sea salt, to taste

Directions:

1. Blend all ingredients in a food processor into a creamy mixture.
2. Serve as a dip for bread, crackers, or any types of vegetables.

Nutrition:

Calories 150

Carbohydrates 23 g

Fats 4 g

Protein 8 g

Greek-style Gigante Beans

Preparation Time: 8 hours 5 minutes

Cooking Time: 10 hours

Servings: 10

Ingredients:

- 12 ounces gigante beans
- 1 can tomatoes with juice, chopped
- 2 stalks celery, diced
- 1 onion, diced
- 4 garlic cloves, minced
- Salt, to taste

Directions:

1. Soak beans in water for 8 hours.
2. Combine drained beans with the remaining ingredients. Stir, and pour water to cover.
3. Cook for 10 hours on low. Season with salt, and serve.

Nutrition:

Calories 63

Carbohydrates 13 g

Fats 2 g

Protein 4 g

Brown Rice & Red Beans & Coconut Milk

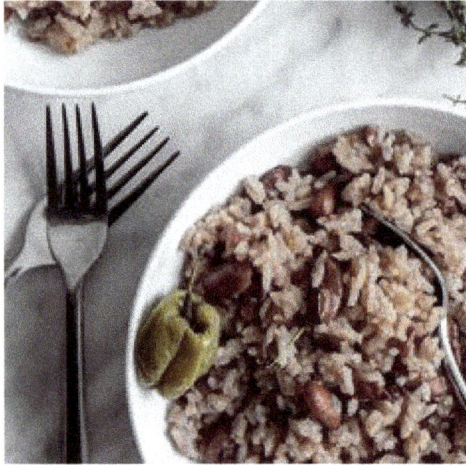

Preparation Time: 10 minutes

Cooking Time: 1 hour

Servings: 6

Ingredients:

- 2 cups brown rice, uncooked
- 4 cups water
- 1 Tbsp olive oil
- 1 onion, diced
- 3 cloves garlic, minced
- 2 cans red beans
- 1 can coconut milk

Directions:

1. Bring brown rice in water to a boil, then simmer for 30 minutes.
2. Sauté onion in olive oil. Add garlic and cook until golden.
3. Mix the onions and garlic, beans, and coconut milk into the rice. Simmer for 15 minutes.
4. Serve hot.

Nutrition:

Calories 280

Carbohydrates 49 g

Fats 3 g

Protein 8 g

Black-Eyed Peas with Herns

Preparation Time: 10 minutes

Cooking Time: 1 hour

Servings: 8

Ingredients:

- 2 cans no-sodium black-eyed beans
- ½ cup extra-virgin olive oil
- 1 cup parsley, chopped
- 4 green onions, sliced
- 2 carrots, grated
- 2 Tbsp tomato paste
- 2 cups water
- Salt, pepper, to taste

Directions:

1. Drain the beans, reserve the liquid.
2. Sauté beans, parsley, onions, and carrots in oil for 3 minutes.
3. Add remaining ingredients, 2 cups reserved beans liquid, and water.
4. Cook for 30 minutes.
5. Season with salt, pepper and serve.

Nutrition:

Calories 230

Carbohydrates 23 g

Fats 15 g

Protein 11 g

Snacks for Morning and Afternoon
Nori Snack Rolls

Preparation Time: 5 Minutes

Cooking Time: 10 Minutes

Servings: 4 Rolls

Ingredients

- 2 tablespoons almond, cashew, peanut, or other nut butter
- 2 tablespoons tamari, or soy sauce
- 4 standard nori sheets
- 1 mushroom, sliced
- 1 tablespoon pickled ginger
- ½ cup grated carrots
-

Directions

1. Preheat the oven to 350°F.
2. Mix together the nut butter and tamari until smooth and very thick. Lay out a nori sheet, rough side up, the long way.
3. Spread a thin line of the tamari mixture on the far end of the nori sheet, from side to side. Lay the

mushroom slices, ginger, and carrots in a line at the other end (the end closest to you).

4. Fold the vegetables inside the nori, rolling toward the tahini mixture, which will seal the roll. Repeat to make 4 rolls.
5. Put on a baking sheet and bake for 8 to 10 minutes, or until the rolls are slightly browned and crispy at the ends. Let the rolls cool for a few minutes, then slice each roll into 3 smaller pieces.

Per Serving (1 roll) Calories: 79; Total fat: 5g; Carbs: 6g; Fiber: 2g; Protein: 4g

Kale Chips

Preparation Time: 5 Minutes

Cooking Time: 25 Minutes

Servings: 2

Ingredients

1 large bunch kale

1 tablespoon extra-virgin olive oil

½ teaspoon chipotle powder

½ teaspoon smoked paprika

¼ teaspoon salt

Directions

1. Preheat the oven to 275ºF.
2. Line a large baking sheet with parchment paper. In a large bowl, stem the kale and tear it into bite-size pieces. Add the olive oil, chipotle powder, smoked paprika, and salt.
3. Toss the kale with tongs or your hands, coating each piece well.
4. Spread the kale over the parchment paper in a single layer.

5. Bake for 25 minutes, turning halfway through, until crisp.

6. Cool for 10 to 15 minutes before dividing and storing in 2 airtight containers.

Nutrition: Calories: 144; Fat: 7g; Protein: 5g; Carbohydrates: 18g; Fiber: 3g; Sugar: 0g; Sodium: 363mg

Savory Roasted Chickpeas

Preparation Time: 5 Minutes

Cooking Time: 25 Minutes

Servings: 1 Cup

Ingredients

- 1 (14-ounce) can chickpeas, rinsed and drained, or 1½ cups cooked
- 2 tablespoons tamari, or soy sauce
- 1 tablespoon nutritional yeast
- 1 teaspoon smoked paprika, or regular paprika
- 1 teaspoon onion powder
- ½ teaspoon garlic powder

Directions

1. Preheat the oven to 400°F.
2. Toss the chickpeas with all the other ingredients, and spread them out on a baking sheet. Bake for 20 to 25 minutes, tossing halfway through.
3. Bake these at a lower temperature, until fully dried and crispy, if you want to keep them longer.

4. You can easily double the batch, and if you dry them out they will keep about a week in an airtight container.

Per Serving (¼ cup) Calories: 121; Total fat: 2g; Carbs: 20g; Fiber: 6g; Protein: 8g

Savory Seed Crackers

Preparation Time: 5 Minutes

Cooking Time: 50 Minutes

Servings: 20 Crackers

Ingredients

- ¾ cup pumpkin seeds (pepitas)
- ½ cup sunflower seeds
- ½ cup sesame seeds
- ¼ cup chia seeds
- 1 teaspoon minced garlic (about 1 clove)
- 1 teaspoon tamari or soy sauce
- 1 teaspoon vegan Worcestershire sauce
- ½ teaspoon ground cayenne pepper
- ½ teaspoon dried oregano
- ½ cup water
-

Directions

1. Preheat the oven to 325ºF.
2. Line a rimmed baking sheet with parchment paper.
3. In a large bowl, combine the pumpkin seeds, sunflower seeds, sesame seeds, chia seeds, garlic,

tamari, Worcestershire sauce, cayenne, oregano, and water.

4. Transfer to the prepared baking sheet, spreading out to all sides.

5. Bake for 25 minutes. Remove the pan from the oven, and flip the seed "dough" over so the wet side is up. Bake for another 20 to 25 minutes, until the sides are browned.

6. Cool completely before breaking up into 20 pieces. Divide evenly among 4 glass jars and close tightly with lids.

Per Serving (5 crackers): Calories: 339; Fat: 29g; Protein: 14g; Carbohydrates: 17g; Fiber: 8g; Sugar: 1g; Sodium: 96mg

Lemon Coconut Cilantro Rolls

Preparation Time: 30 Minutes • Chill Time: 30 Minutes
Servings: 16 Pieces

Ingredients

- ½ cup fresh cilantro, chopped
- 1 cup sprouts (clover, alfalfa)
- 1 garlic clove, pressed
- 2 tablespoons ground Brazil nuts or almonds
- 2 tablespoons flaked coconut
- 1 tablespoon coconut oil
- Pinch cayenne pepper
- Pinch sea salt
- Pinch freshly ground black pepper
- Zest and juice of 1 lemon
- 2 tablespoons ground flaxseed
- 1 to 2 tablespoons water
- 2 whole-wheat wraps, or corn wraps

Directions

1. Put everything but the wraps in a food processor and pulse to combine. Or combine the ingredients

in a large bowl. Add the water, if needed, to help the mix come together.

2. Spread the mixture out over each wrap, roll it up, and place it in the fridge for 30 minutes to set.

3. Remove the rolls from the fridge and slice each into 8 pieces to serve as appetizers or sides with a soup or stew.

4. Get the best flavor by buying whole raw Brazil nuts or almonds, toasting them lightly in a dry skillet or toaster oven, and then grinding them in a coffee grinder.

Per Serving (1 piece) Calories: 66; Total fat: 4g; Carbs: 6g; Fiber: 1g; Protein: 2g

Tamari Almonds

Preparation Time: 5 Minutes

Cooking Time: 15 Minutes

Servings: 8

Ingredients

- 1 pound raw almonds
- 3 tablespoons tamari or soy sauce
- 2 tablespoons extra-virgin olive oil
- 1 tablespoon nutritional yeast
- 1 to 2 teaspoons chili powder, to taste

Directions

1. Preheat the oven to 400ºF.
2. Line a baking sheet with parchment paper.
3. In a medium bowl, combine the almonds, tamari, and olive oil until well coated.
4. Spread the almonds on the prepared baking sheet and roast for 10 to 15 minutes, until browned.
5. Cool for 10 minutes, then season with the nutritional yeast and chili powder.
6. Transfer to a glass jar and close tightly with a lid.

Nutrition: Calories: 364; Fat: 32g; Protein: 13g; Carbohydrates: 13g; Fiber: 7g; Sugar: 3g; Sodium: 381mg

Tempeh Taco Bites

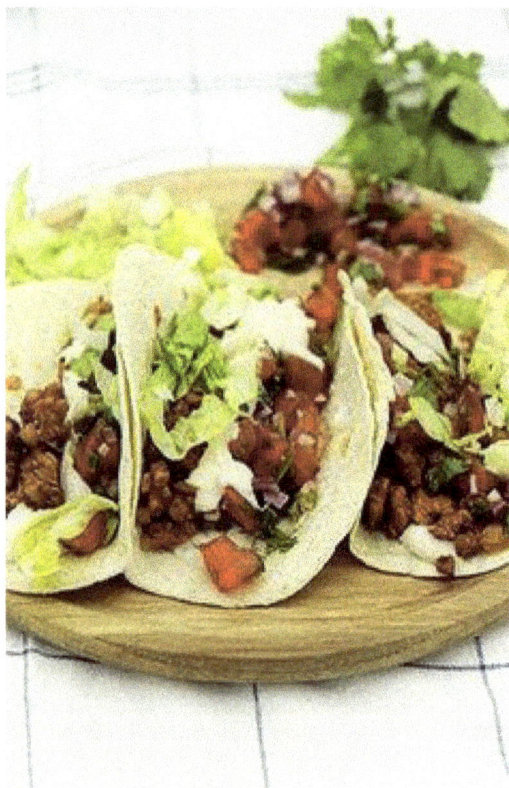

PREPARATION TIME: 5 MINUTES

Cooking Time: 45 MINUTES

Servings: 3 Dozen

Ingredients

- 8 ounces tempeh
- 3 tablespoons soy sauce
- 2 teaspoons ground cumin

- 1 teaspoon chili powder
- 1 teaspoon dried oregano
- 1 tablespoon olive oil
- 1/2 cup finely minced onion
- 2 garlic cloves, minced
- Salt and freshly ground black pepper
- 2 tablespoons tomato paste
- 1 chipotle chile in adobo, finely minced
- 1/4 cup hot water or vegetable broth, homemade or store-bought, plus more if needed
- 36 phyllo pastry cups, thawed
- 1/2 cup basic guacamole, homemade or store-bought
- 18 ripe cherry tomatoes, halved

Directions

1. In a medium saucepan of simmering water, cook the tempeh for 30 minutes. Drain well, then finely mince and place it in a bowl. Add the soy sauce, cumin, chili powder, and oregano. Mix well and set aside.

2. In a medium skillet, heat the oil over medium heat. Add the onion, cover, and cook for 5 minutes. Stir in the garlic, then add the tempeh mixture and

cook, stirring, for 2 to 3 minutes. Season with salt and pepper to taste. Set aside.

3. In a small bowl, combine the tomato paste, chipotle, and the hot water or broth. Return tempeh mixture to heat and in stir tomato-chile mixture and cook for 10 to 15 minutes, stirring occasionally, until the liquid is absorbed.

4. The mixture should be fairly dry, but if it begins to stick to the pan, add a little hotter water, 1 tablespoon at a time. Taste, adjusting seasonings if necessary. Remove from the heat.

5. To assemble, fill the phyllo cups to the top with the tempeh filling, using about 2 teaspoons of filling in each. Top with a dollop of guacamole and a cherry tomato half and serve.

Mushroom Croustades

Preparation Time: 10 Minutes

Cooking Time: 10 Minutes

Servings: 12 Croustades

Ingredients

- 12 thin slices whole-grain bread
- 1 tablespoon olive oil, plus more for brushing bread
- 2 medium shallots, chopped
- 2 garlic cloves, minced
- 12 ounces white mushrooms, chopped
- 1/4 cup chopped fresh parsley
- 1 teaspoon dried thyme
- 1 tablespoon soy sauce

Directions

1. Preheat the oven to 400°F. Using a 3-inch round pastry cutter or a drinking glass, cut a circle from each bread slice. Brush the bread circles with oil and press them firmly but gently into a mini-muffin tin. Bake until the bread is toasted, about 10 minutes.
2. Meanwhile, in a large skillet, heat the 1 tablespoon oil over medium heat. Add the shallots, garlic, and

mushrooms and sauté for 5 minutes to soften the vegetables. Stir in the parsley, thyme, and soy sauce and cook until the liquid is absorbed, about 5 minutes longer. Spoon the mushroom mixture into the croustade cups and return to the oven for 3 to 5 minutes to heat through. Serve warm.

Stuffed Cherry Tomatoes

Preparation Time: 15 Minutes

Cooking Time: 0 Minutes

Servings: 6

Ingredients

- 2 pints cherry tomatoes, tops removed and centers scooped out
- 2 avocados, mashed
- juice of 1 lemon
- ½ red bell pepper, minced
- 4 green onions (white and green parts), finely minced
- 1 tablespoon minced fresh tarragon
- pinch of sea salt

Directions

1. Place the cherry tomatoes open-side up on a platter.
2. In a small bowl, combine the avocado, lemon juice, bell pepper, scallions, tarragon, and salt.
3. Stir until well combined. Scoop into the cherry tomatoes and serve immediately.

Spicy Black Bean Dip

Preparation Time: 10 Minutes

Cooking Time: 0 Minutes

Servings: 2 Cups

Ingredients

- 1 (14-ounce) can black beans, drained and rinsed, or 1½ cups cooked
- Zest and juice of 1 lime
- 1 tablespoon tamari, or soy sauce
- ¼ cup water
- ¼ cup fresh cilantro, chopped
- 1 teaspoon ground cumin
- Pinch cayenne pepper

Directions

1. Put the beans in a food processor (best choice) or blender, along with the lime zest and juice, tamari, and about ¼ cup of water.
2. Blend until smooth, then blend in the cilantro, cumin, and cayenne.
3. If you don't have a blender or prefer a different consistency, simply transfer it to a bowl once the

beans have been puréed and stir in the spices, instead of forcing the blender.

Per Serving (1 cup) Calories: 190; Total fat: 1g; Carbs: 35g; Fiber: 12g; Protein: 13g

French Onion Pastry Puffs

Preparation Time: 10 Minutes

Cooking Time: 35 Minutes - Makes 24 Puffs

Ingredients

- 2 tablespoons olive oil
- 2 medium onions, thinly sliced
- 1 garlic clove, minced
- 1 teaspoon chopped fresh rosemary
- Salt and freshly ground black pepper
- 1 tablespoon capers
- 1 sheet frozen vegan puff pastry, thawed
- 18 pitted black olives, quartered

Directions

1. In a medium skillet, heat the oil over medium heat. Add the onions and garlic, season with rosemary and salt and pepper to taste. Cover and cook until very soft, stirring occasionally, about 20 minutes. Stir in the capers and set aside.

2. Preheat the oven to 400°F. Roll out the puff pastry and cut into 2- to 3-inch circles using a lightly

floured pastry cutter or drinking glass. You should get about 2 dozen circles.

3. Arrange the pastry circles on baking sheets and top each with a heaping teaspoon of onion mixture, patting down to smooth the top.

4. Top with 3 olive quarters, arranged decoratively— either like flower petals emanating from the center or parallel to each other like 3 bars.

5. Bake until pastry is puffed and golden brown, about 15 minutes. Serve hot.

Cheezy Cashew–Roasted Red Pepper Toasts

Preparation Time: 15 Minutes

Cooking Time: 0 Minutes

Servings: 16 To 24 Toasts

Ingredients

- 2 jarred roasted red peppers
- 1 cup unsalted cashews
- 1/4 cup water
- 1 tablespoon soy sauce
- 2 tablespoons chopped green onions
- 1/4 cup nutritional yeast
- 2 tablespoons balsamic vinegar
- 2 tablespoons olive oil

Directions

1. Use canapé or cookie cutters to cut the bread into desired shapes about 2 inches wide. If you don't have a cutter, use a knife to cut the bread into squares, triangles, or rectangles. You should get 2 to 4 pieces out of each slice of bread. Toast the bread and set aside to cool.

2. Coarsely chop 1 red pepper and set aside. Cut the remaining pepper into thin strips or decorative shapes and set aside for garnish.

3. In a blender or food processor, grind the cashews to a fine powder. Add the water and soy sauce and process until smooth. Add the chopped red pepper and puree. Add the green onions, nutritional yeast, vinegar, and oil and process until smooth and well blended.

4. Spread a spoonful of the pepper mixture onto each of the toasted bread pieces and top decoratively with the reserved pepper strips. Arrange on a platter or tray and serve.

Baked Potato Chips

Preparation Time: 10 Minutes

Cooking Time: 30 Minutes

Servings: 4

Ingredients

- 1 large Russet potato
- 1 teaspoon paprika
- ½ teaspoon garlic salt
- ¼ teaspoon vegan sugar
- ¼ teaspoon onion powder
- ¼ teaspoon chipotle powder or chili powder
- ⅛ teaspoon salt
- ⅛ teaspoon ground mustard
- ⅛ teaspoon ground cayenne pepper
- 1 teaspoon canola oil
- ⅛ teaspoon liquid smoke

Directions

1. Wash and peel the potato. Cut into thin, 1/10-inch slices (a mandoline slicer or the slicer blade in a food processor is helpful for consistently sized slices).

2. Fill a large bowl with enough very cold water to cover the potato. Transfer the potato slices to the bowl and soak for 20 minutes.

3. Preheat the oven to 400ºF. Line a baking sheet with parchment paper.

4. In a small bowl, combine the paprika, garlic salt, sugar, onion powder, chipotle powder, salt, mustard, and cayenne.

5. Drain and rinse the potato slices and pat dry with a paper towel.

6. Transfer to a large bowl.

7. Add the canola oil, liquid smoke, and spice mixture to the bowl. Toss to coat.

8. Transfer the potatoes to the prepared baking sheet.

9. Bake for 15 minutes. Flip the chips over and bake for 15 minutes longer, until browned. Transfer the chips to 4 storage containers or large glass jars.

10.   Let cool before closing the lids tightly.

Nutrition: Calories: 89; Fat: 1g; Protein: 2g; Carbohydrates: 18g; Fiber: 2g; Sugar: 1g; Sodium: 65mg

www.ingramcontent.com/pod-product-compliance
Lightning Source LLC
Chambersburg PA
CBHW050755030426
42336CB00012B/1829